Simple Steps To Yonanas Making

A Straight Forward Guide To The Best Yonanas Recipes To Make At Home For Your Family

Laura Salinas

Table Of Contents

Introduction

Yonanas Frozen Treat Maker is a kitchen gadget that turns any fruit into a delicious soft-serve style treat that can be made at home with no added sugar.

People want to find ways to eat healthier and make their favorite sweet treats more nutritious. Yonanas Frozen Treat Maker is a kitchen gadget that turns any fruit into a delicious soft-serve style treat without the need for added sugar or additives. The Yonanas was invented by Anthony Sosnick while he was watching his health improve after adopting a vegan diet and learning about the benefits of raw food. He got the idea for Yonanas when trying to create healthy frozen desserts but not wanting to use cream and other ingredients whose health benefits he found questionable.

Yonanas had been a popular to-do item for many years, and Sosnick was prompted to pursue the idea through Kickstarter. The Yonanas Kickstarter achieved worldwide press coverage and caught the attention of investors. The sales pitch for the idea was simple: "So, sugars are bad, right?"

The Yonanas is simple to use. It replaces the need for an ice cream maker and uses frozen fruits as the base for the frozen dessert. All it takes is a frozen banana and fruit of your choice (berries, mango, pineapple, etc.), and presto—you have a healthy treat. The Yonanas works by blending fresh or frozen fruits into a smoothie-like texture. Customers can choose to add additional ingredients such as chocolate chips or nuts before blending for a more flavorful experience. The Yonanas has no added sugar and uses no artificial ingredients for this same reason. Sosnick has built a company, Yonanas LLC, to produce the Yonanas as well as provide information and ideas on making healthy treats at home. The Yonanas frozen treat maker will be available at nationwide retailers this spring—including Target, Walmart, and Bed Bath & Beyond in addition to Amazon and IndiHome online stores.

Health Benefits of Yonanas Dessert

There are health benefits to using Yonanas Frozen Treat Makers, and they are as follows:

1. First, you can use Yonanas to make raw frozen fruit treats.

2. Secondly, you don't need to add sugar, as the natural sweetness of the fruit is preserved.

3. Thirdly, you preserve the vitamins and nutrients that are found in fresh fruits.

4. You can control the portion size of your frozen treat by adding more or less fruit into your blend.

5. You can use your Yonanas to make healthy recipes, such as desserts and frozen treats, with no added sugar.

6. Lastly, you can relish the taste of your favorite frozen treat without worrying about any negative side effects.

In addition to its benefits, Yonanas Frozen Treat Maker helps people to maintain a healthy lifestyle at home and at work while providing an affordable and convenient solution for making healthy desserts and snacks quickly with minimum fuss.

Why You Need This Book

This book contains basic information about Yonanas Frozen Treat Maker that everyone should have to make the most of the product. It is written in an easy-to-understand language that will help you to solve problems or troubles when using Yonanas Frozen Treat Maker. Then you will save both time and money and enjoy healthy treats without additives and preservatives such as refined sugar.

The purpose of this book is to make your life easier by providing you with essential information, from basic tools needed for Yonanas Frozen Treat Maker to technical issues such as cleaning and storage. Also, it covers nutritional information about Yonanas Frozen Treat Maker ingredients because they affect overall health and safety, which is vital for everyone today.

Other than the basics of Yonanas Frozen Treat Maker, this book also contains recipes and additional information on ingredients and their health benefits. These recipes will provide you with more information on Yonanas Frozen Treat Maker features and how to use them in the most efficient way, which may not be covered by the manufacturer's manual.

Presently there are many frozen dessert machines on the market. However, Yonanas Frozen Treat Maker is different from other products due to its ability to make delicious frozen treats from a variety of ingredients. This book will show you how to choose, store, and clean Yonanas Frozen Treat Maker properly. You will also find out why it is important to follow the manufacturer's instructions and tips on how to avoid common mistakes that can lead to negative results.

So, let us get started.

CHAPTER 1:

Why Choose a Yonanas Frozen Healthy Dessert Maker

Everything these days is on a fast-track. We want convenient, quick, and easy—fast food, grocery delivery service, overnight shipping.

Sure, ice cream makers and food processors have a place in our kitchen, but sometimes the time just doesn't exist for multi-step, long process recipes. Get a Yonanas Healthy Dessert Maker® and get instant dessert.

It's a lightweight, all-in-one-piece model, which makes it super easy to store, clean, and travel with. Everything can be attached, which means no loose pieces will be falling all over the place when it's pulled out of storage or off the shelf. The important parts are all dishwasher safe, so only limited scrubbing is required. Make dessert and instantly enjoy it instead of spending time cleaning up and staring at the clock, waiting for the moment it's finally frozen enough to eat.

Enjoy instant ice creams and sorbets, frozen cakes, pies and popsicles, and even some non-dessert dishes like hummus and mashed potatoes.

How to Use Your Yonanas Frozen Treat Maker
Easy Peasy.

- All you do is feed frozen fruit and other ingredients of your choice into the chute.

- Turn on the machine and press down with the plastic plunger when the chute is full.

- The product is a creamy frozen treat, instant ice creams, and frozen yogurt.

How It Compares to Other Machines

With the market as saturated with blenders and ice cream makers, it can be hard to make a decision about which merchandise to purchase. Educating yourself about other products and how they stack up against the Yonanas Healthy Dessert Maker® is the best solution.

Ice Cream Makers

Perfect for making ice cream. This may seem obvious, but this is what small appliances like the Cuisinart ICE-100 were precisely created to do. Making your ice cream at home can be beneficial since you can control the ingredients. You can control dietary restrictions like dairy and opt for almond or coconut milk, and you can cut on the total of sugar that goes into your dessert. Some ice cream makers are 100% automatic and come with self-freezing bowls, yielding instant gratification with ready to eat ice cream. However, ice cream makers come at a cost. Most of these appliances pack quite a punch to your pocketbook and are incredibly difficult to clean and maintain.

Frozen Dessert Makers

There are a few brands of dessert makers similar to the Yonanas Healthy Dessert Maker®. The Magic Dessert Bullet® and Big Boss Swirlo® are the most comparable. But what is the real difference between the brands? Not much. Power and dimensions are the biggest difference on paper. The Magic Bullet is the winner when it comes to power. With 350 Watts, it is the most powerful of the three, followed by the Yonanas Healthy Dessert Maker® with 200 Watts and the Big Boss Swirlo® with only 130 Watts. Why is this important? Because when grinding up frozen fruit, you want the machine to be able to handle it without shutting down. The dimensions also vary just slightly. For the most part, the machines look similar; all have plungers and chutes, are made of plastic, BPA-free, and dishwasher safe. While the function of a particular device might suit you better, this is something you won't know until you've purchased one and tried it out. The Yonanas Healthy Dessert Maker® is currently the most expensive, followed by the Magic Bullet Dessert Bullet® and the Big Boss Swirlo®.

Pros & Cons

We consider the Yonanas Healthy Dessert Maker® to be a fantastic choice for your household frozen dessert appliance. We want you to consider all your selections. Make informed decisions. Here are some Pros and Cons of the machine.

Pros

- **Healthy:** Frozen fruits make this a healthy option. Less sugar and dairy-free, if you want. You choose your fixings. You regulate what goes into the machine. There are so many selections, both healthy and not so healthy. The ingredients and combinations are endless.

- **Super easy to use:** Fill the chute, press down on the plastic plunger to send ingredients through the chute, and enjoy. It is that easy. 1-2-3.

- **Multipurpose:** Dishwasher safe. Even though you have to take apart and rinse the individual pieces, you can quickly pop them into the dishwasher.

- **Lightweight:** The machine itself is super lightweight and very easy to move around. You can take it to a friend's house or an event so easily.

- **It's fun to experiment:** This is the number one reason to purchase the Yonanas Healthy Dessert Maker®. It's fun. The possibilities are endless. You can just toss in whatever sweet treats you have lying around your home and have an instant creamy dessert.

Cons

- **Noisy:** While this machine is not much stronger than a blender, many users have mentioned that it is really loud. The Yonanas Elite Frozen Healthy Dessert Maker® is said to be a bit quieter.

- **Not a breeze to clean:** Dishwasher safe doesn't mean just pop the whole thing into the dishwasher. Frozen fruits can be tricky and get sticky if not rinsed right away. Unscrewing the parts and rinsing them under warm water or soaking them for a while can help cut back on the cleaning issues many users complain about.

CHAPTER 2:

Getting to Know Your Yonanas Healthy Dessert Maker

For foodies, appliances can turn out to be best friends or enemies. They're very much like people. The more you get to know your device, the more likely you are to fall in love with it, and the more you want to see it, spend time with it, do new and exciting things with it. So, get to know how your Yonanas Healthy Dessert Maker®. I guarantee you will be delighted when you discover all the awesome it has to offer.

Yonanas Healthy Dessert Maker® Accessories Included

Here's what comes in the box. Make sure it's all here before you start making awesome treats.

- **Base:** This is the heart and soul of the machine. It houses the motor and has an electrical cord
- **Chute:** This is where all the ingredients are inserted. It also covers the blade
- **Plunger:** Used to press down the food when the chute gets full
- **Blade Cone:** The actual blade
- **Gasket:** Plastic that goes under the blade to prevent leakage
- **Bottom cap:** Screws everything together and makes the machine one nice, connected piece of equipment.

Other Accessories Not Included

- **Pie pan:** Pie and cake recipes call for a pie pan, so if you don't have one, pick one up. 9-inch.
- **Popsicle trays:** You can make your own with Dixie cups and popsicle sticks, but it is much easier to purchase some

inexpensive plastic ones that can be reused. Buy different sizes yielding a different number of servings. You never know how many people you will be feeding with your popsicles.

- **Ice cube trays:** Some recipes will make cute little bite-sized treats. Ice cube trays are used to freeze them in, so mix it up and try some fun shapes.

- **Small mixing bowls:** Having all your ingredients lined up and ready to go is a must. The machine moves quickly, so have some small bowls available will all your ingredients measured out.

- **Stainless steel bowls:** Some recipes call for stainless steel bowls for easy heating. You will need this if you pick to try those recipes. There is no acceptable substitute.

- **Measuring cups and spoons:** Everything is measured out. So even though this is not an exact science, you will want to get in the general area of correct measurements.

Assembly

1. Remove all parts from the plastic.
2. Insert the rubber gasket into the hard-plastic bottom cap. Be sure to put the bottom part of the gasket (larger part) into the top part of the cap.
3. The blade cone turns on top of the gasket, making one piece.
4. Screw the one piece into the plastic chute. The bottom cap and chute will screw together, but be sure it is evenly in place. This will also create one piece.
5. Take the cute and fit it into the machine base. Turn counterclockwise until it clicks.
6. You should have one piece with no loose parts.

CHAPTER 3:

How To

How to Adjust Recipes for the Yonanas Healthy Dessert Maker

You can adjust almost any frozen dessert recipe to fit your Yonanas Healthy Dessert Maker®. Whether it's ice cream, healthy dessert, frozen fruit treats, frozen yogurt, popsicles, or even frozen pies and cakes you're after, this little machine can do it all. There is just a limited thing to keep in mind when converting recipes.

Liquids

Limit the amount of liquid you use. The chute is open straight through, from top to bottom. The Yonanas Healthy Dessert Maker® is not a juicer, so if you put in a liquid by itself, it will run right out. Try mixing the liquids with other ingredients and alternate adding ingredients. Add some solids before and after the fluids. If it is necessary to use liquids, try freezing it for a little bit until it becomes slushy. Everything comes out super creamy, so you shouldn't need a whole lot of liquid anyway.

Timing

Most of the actual work is just running ingredients through the chute. This is a quick process, usually only taking a few minutes. It goes very quickly, so be sure to have everything you need set out in bowls so you don't have to scramble to feed in the next ingredient. Soft serve, frozen yogurt, and ice cream take only minutes to complete but keep in mind that if you are making popsicles or frozen desserts like cakes and pies, you will still need to budget 3-4 hours of freeze time.

Do Not Use Ice

While it is okay to use frozen ingredients, like fruit or juice concentrate, it is never okay to use ice. The chute is relatively small, and the blades are shaped and housed differently than a blender or food processor. If you need to pre-freeze ingredients like milk or yogurt, just be sure it is only frozen to a slushy consistency and not rock hard. Using ice or other extremely hard, frozen solids will likely damage your machine.

Non-Dessert Recipes

When making non-dessert recipes like hummus or mashed potatoes, be sure that your ingredients are always precooked—nothing raw, especially eggs. Since you won't be using frozen fruits, your ingredients like potatoes should be boiled, not too soft, though, and slightly cooled. You will need something solid, but not too hard, that can be easily pushed through the chute and made into a creamy texture. You will be a Yonanas expert soon, so apply all the same rules, like alternating ingredients and limiting your liquids, to your non-dessert recipes.

How to Operate Your Yonanas Healthy Dessert Maker

Your Yonanas Healthy Dessert Maker® is super easy to use. Every recipe, no matter what the ingredients, follows the same steps.

1. Set out all ingredients. The machine moves fast, so be sure to have all your ingredients measured out and into bowls for a smooth process.
2. Place a bowl under the chute to clasp all your treats.
3. Turn on the machine.
4. Alternate adding ingredients to the chute until it is full; make sure to sandwich liquids in between solids, so they don't run straight through the chute.
5. Press down with the plastic plunger, pushing ingredients through the chute.
6. Repeat steps 4 and 5 until all fixings are used.

Minutes later, you will have a delicious treat to enjoy. Be sure to completely disassembled and clean the appliance after each use.

How to Store Your Soft-Serve Dessert

If you have a crazy amount of self-control and don't enjoy your frozen snacks immediately after making them, we envy you. Treats can usually be stored up to 2 or 3 weeks in the freezer. You can purchase freezer bags or use containers.

Freezer Bags

Be sure your baggies are "freezer" baggies. This seems obvious but is often accidentally overlooked, and no one likes freezer burn. If you choose to use freezer bags, all you need to do is toss your treats inside and zip them up. Make sure they are completely frozen, so they don't stick together.

Storage Containers

You can also use containers to store your treats. Be sure to layer with parchment paper, so they don't stick together. Items stored in containers are usually more tightly packed than when stored in freezer bags and sometimes get stuck together.

Cleaning and Disassembling Your Yonanas Healthy Dessert Maker®

So now you have a fabulous frozen dessert to enjoy, but don't forget to clean your machine immediately. If you do not have time to clean it right away, at least rinse it under some warm water. This helps all the fruit to wash off and makes for an easier clean up later. Rinsing helps to prevent fruit from sticking and any future scrubbing.

1. Turn the chute clockwise until it comes loose.
2. Remove the plunger from the chute.
3. Unscrew the bottom cap and blade cone. Be careful as the blade is sharp!
4. Separate the rubber gasket, bottom cap, and blade cone.
5. Rinse all pieces, except the base, under warm water. You can use a scrub brush to remove particles stuck in the blades or corners of the gasket and bottom cap.
6. Wipe the base with a damp cloth. DO NOT RINSE OR SUBMERGE IN WATER. The base has an electrical cord. It should never be submerged in water.
7. Put all parts, not the base, into the dishwasher.

You're ready for more Yonanas fun!

CHAPTER 4:

Topping/Additives Guide

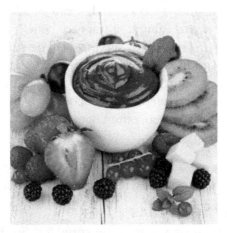

Nut Butters

Nut kinds of butter are always a nice flavor that can be added to many frozen treats. They can be used in a couple of ways. First, you can run a few tablespoons through the Yonanas Healthy Dessert Maker® along with the other ingredients. This will help to blend well with the other ingredients and give more of an overall flavor. Be sure not to add more than three tablespoons as it could clog up the chute and blades. You can also hand swirl the nut butter in after. Just dollop the butter into the frozen treats and swirl with a spoon. This option gives a burst of flavor. Some great options would be apple butter, peanut butter, almond butter, or Nutella.

Milk

When adding milk, it is crucial not to use too much. A few tablespoons can go a long way add flavor and a creamy texture. Unless the recipe calls for more, two tablespoons are usually enough. Liquid runs right through the chute, so be sure to put a solid in first. You can always partially freeze the milk to create a slushy texture. This will help keep the liquid from running out. Besides obvious dairy milk, try almond milk, soy milk, or coconut milk. They come in all types of tastes like vanilla, chocolate, or strawberry, and be purchased sweetened or unsweetened.

Yogurt

Yogurt can be fun. Many recipes already call for its use, but don't feel like you need to use the flavor the recipe calls for. With so many different brands and so many different flavors, there is no reason not to experiment. Since yogurt is a soft solid, it can be added to the machine as-is with ease, but try freezing it in mini-ice cube trays or in spoonfuls on parchment paper. The frozen servings will be even easier to plunge into the machine with the frozen fruit. Greek yogurt will yield a thicker texture than regular yogurt, but it will also have more of a bite to it. If you are trying to be dairy-free, opt for coconut yogurt. They have Greek coconut yogurt and regular coconut yogurt as well.

Fruits

Double up on the fruit action. Chop fruits, or use their natural juices as garnishes. Fresh fruit would be a nice compliment to a frozen fruit treat.

Frinkles and Sprinkles

The little kid in all of us wants some sprinkles. So, honor your inner child and give yourself a nice tablespoon of rainbow or chocolate sprinkles! Too much sugar for your taste? Yonanas makes little bags of awesome toppings called "Frinkles." These are freeze-dried fruits that look like sprinkles. They come in flavors like Berry Blast and Tropical Fruit.

Cookie Dough

Find some great cookie dough! Add it on top of any recipe for an added treat. Be sure to use vegan cookie dough, so you don't consume uncooked eggs.

Sauces

Sauce it up. Don't be afraid to add some strawberry, chocolate, or caramel sauce to your frozen treats. You can add a tablespoon or 2 to the chute with the other ingredients for an overall flavor or drizzle some sauce on top of the finished product.

Soda

Have afloat. Toss some ice cream or frozen bites in something carbonated. Don't stop at a root beer or coke float, but try other flavors like cream soda, sarsaparilla, or something that will complement the flavor of your treat.

Nuts or Coconut Flakes

Garnish your fro-yo or ice cream with roasted, toasted, or fresh nuts or flakes. Pistachios, almonds, cashews, walnuts, macadamia nuts, peanuts, or coconut are some great choices to sprinkle on top of any frozen dessert. It adds a new flavor and a different texture.

Cookies

Crumble your favorite cookie and add as a topping or add some during your creation process. Add some crunch to your creamy. Oreos, gingersnaps, vanilla wafers, and chocolate chip cookies are always great options, but we'll let you choose your favorite.

CHAPTER 5:

Texture Guide and Pantry Stocking Guide

Texture Guide

Not all frozen treats are created equal. Different desserts are made with different ingredients, thus yielding different textures and flavors. Here is a cheat sheet to help you decide which one suits you best.

Ice Cream

Cool and creamy, this dessert is usually made with milk. It also typically contains sugar or corn syrup for a very sweet flavor.

Sorbet

If the fruit is your thing, then sorbet should be your go-to frozen treat. The texture is rough and somewhat icy, as sorbet is almost always dairy-free. Flavors are refreshing and zestier tasting than creamy.

Sherbet

Not to get confused with sorbet, Sherbet typically contains dairy. The taste is similar to sorbet in that it is refreshing and fruity, but sherbet will have a creamier texture and flavor because of the dairy content. Keep in mind that nondairy milk will yield equally smooth results, so don't rule sherbet out completely if you're going for a dairy-free dessert.

Popsicle

Popsicles aren't always frozen, icy treats; some can have a fudgy or creamy texture. Most popsicles are frozen using popsicle trays with sticks, but popsicle bites are becoming a new trend. By using ice cube trays with no sticks, popsicle recipes can be transformed into bite-sized treats in fun shapes. The bites are also easier to transport in baggies or containers.

Gelato

Rich. Decadent. Elegant. All words that accurately describe gelato. It is almost always higher in sugar and will have a softer texture as it does not freeze completely.

Frozen Yogurt

Made with, you guessed it! Yogurt. Whether it is Greek yogurt, regular yogurt, low-fat, or coconut yogurt, you can bet on yogurt being in your, well, frozen yogurt. While sugar is sometimes added, this frozen treat has a little bit of a bite or hint of sour to it because yogurt is the main ingredient—fruit and chocolate complement almost any fro-yo flavor.

Pantry Stocking Guide

The possibilities with your Yonanas Healthy Dessert Maker® are virtually endless. The good news is that many recipes use the same or similar ingredients. You can always go ahead and freeze your treats.

Since many of these ingredients come frozen or are non-perishable, it makes sense to purchase them in bulk.

List of the most mentioned ingredients in this book. Use it as a guide for your shopping list.

- **Sugar:** You can always use natural sweeteners, but if you choose to use sugar, try to find a quick dissolve, superfine sugar. Regular sugar can also be run through a food processor to make it finer. It makes for a less grainy texture.

- **Honey, agave nectar, or stevia:** Natural sweeteners are a go-to for healthy desserts. The taste isn't changed that much, and they are low-glycemic. The honey and nectar can also create a nice binding agent for some recipes.

- **Frozen Bananas:** Buy them in bulk, like they are going out of style. Most recipes will call for a banana or 2. You can buy pre-sliced frozen bananas in very large quantities.

- **Cheetah spotted bananas:** Stock up on fresh bananas too. The cheetah spotted ones are the sweetest. Be sure they are "cheetah spotted" and not completely brown. Peel and slice into ¼ inch thick pieces. Store in a freezer bag or vessel for future use.

- **Frozen fruits:** Every recipe is going to call for some kind of frozen fruit. The possibilities are limitless, so buy any frozen

27 | P a g .

fruit you like. Strawberries, blueberries, raspberries, blackberries, cherries, melons, peaches, pineapples, and mangos are some of the most popular.

- **Fresh fruits:** Buy and freeze your favorites. Pineapples, mangos, peaches, kiwi, and grapes are some of the popular fruits that are difficult to find already frozen. Just buy the fruit fresh, slice into ¼ inch thick pieces and freeze in freezer bags or containers until you're ready to use them.

- **Peanut butter:** Peanut butter can be pretty awesome in frozen treats. Stock up if that's your thing.

- **Nutella:** For decades, everyone's hazelnut favorite.

- **Cocoa powder:** Sweetened or unsweetened, cocoa powder is found in chocolate recipes. A lot goes a long way, plus you can usually find it in an easily sealable container.

- **Milk:** Chose your flavor. Many healthy options are available, like almond, soy, and coconut milk, and come in different flavors. The boxed milk can be found on sale and not refrigerated. You can store these in your pantry until you are ready to use them.

- **Canned coconut milk:** Not to be jumbled with boxed or refrigerated coconut milk. Canned coconut milk separates. The top part is usually a thick layer of what is referred to as "coconut cream," and the bottom part is "coconut milk." All recipes will call for the canned milk to be refrigerated. It is okay to store the can in the fridge before it has been opened.

- **Greek yogurt:** Greek yogurt has a heavier consistency than regular yogurt. This helps for a thicker dessert. Its flavor is also a little bit more tart than regular yogurt. Be sure to buy regular, vanilla, and low-fat or fat-free varieties.

- **Toasted nuts:** Walnuts, pecan, cashews, peanuts. Choose whichever nuts you would like to use. Typically, a garnish.

- **Coconut flakes:** Toasted coconut flakes complement many desserts.

- **Chocolate chips:** Used as a garnish and also as chunks run through the machine. Regular size or minis.

- **Sprinkles:** Rainbow, colored, or chocolate! Jazz up your dessert.

- **Dark chocolate:** Choose bars of dark chocolate. Recipes range from 70%-85%.

- **Cookies:** Pies and cakes use different cookie crumbs for the crust. Graham crackers, Oreos, and gingersnaps are some of the most popular.

- **Canola Oil:** A few tablespoons of canola oil are added to cookie crumbs to make pie crusts.

- **Eggs:** Use large eggs.

- **Pie crusts:** Frozen pie crusts can cut back on prep time.

- **Lemons and limes:** Add a little kick. Many of the refreshing recipes will ask for lemon and lime zest or juice.

- **Extracts:** Vanilla, almond, and peppermint are some of the big ones.

CHAPTER 6:

Taste Hacking Guide

L et's be honest, while smoothies and blended treats can be the easiest to make; things can and do go terribly wrong. Not everything turns out the way it should, resulting in an end product being too bitter, too thin, too thick, or even too sweet (yes, that is actually a thing). Not to worry, here are some simple fixes for your Yonanas Healthy Dessert Maker®.

When It's Too Bitter

While green veggies can be a main component of smoothies, they can also be the main contributor to that unwelcome bitter taste. But don't remove the greens! Try using baby spinach because it has a gentler flavor. Use sweeter fruits.

Try pairing greens with fruits like bananas, pineapples, dates, blueberries, or strawberries. The sweet flavors will complement the bitter greens and make them not as harsh. Stevia, honey, agave nectar, and vanilla are some great natural sweeteners that will help counteract any bitterness, but be careful; a little goes a long way. If a sweet flavor wouldn't be your first choice, opt for some lemon or lime juice. The juice cuts through the bitterness and can create a refreshing, cool taste. Consider adding protein powder too. Not only will it boost protein intake, of course, but the powders come in fun flavors that can add a twist to any treat.

When It's Too Sweet

It happens. Every once in a while, you get a super sweet smoothie. The first fix is if you're adding sugar or other sweeteners, just don't. The smallest amount can add an explosion of flavor. Consider using low-glycemic fruits like blackberries, grapefruits, or avocados. If using milk or other additives, opt for the unsweetened or sugar-free version. And of course, the end-all, be-all, fix-all is to add some lemon or lime juice and get a refreshing burst of flavor instead.

When It's Too Thick

If your smoothies come out too thick, try adding some water, milk, coffee, or juice, but be sure not to add too much. Use less frozen and fresher. Sometimes the frozen fruits can be too thick and hard and not produce enough juice to thin out the smoothie. Next time try alternating liquids and solids, putting liquids in first.

When It's Too Thin

Sometimes they come out too thin. We're going' for smoothies and frozen treats here, folks, not juices! If you run into this super common issue, try using fruits with thick skins. Peaches, mangos, dates, and apricots make perfect thickeners. Bananas, avocados, and Greek yogurt are great too. Alternate the adding of liquids and solids. Add fruits and veggies first.

This prevents all the liquid from pooling. Guar gum and xanthan gum are great options, especially for alcoholic treats, that tend to get runny. Both are gluten-free. They function like gluten and help to bind and create volume. Just like sweeteners, a little of these additives go a long way. Try only using 1/8 of a teaspoon; otherwise, you will have another consistency issue on your hands.

When It's Too Sour

Some desserts are made to be tangy and sour, but then again, too much of anything is never a good thing. Try adding more bananas or other sweeter fruits to help off put the sourness. If the recipe calls for milk or other liquids, trying to add an additional tablespoon, just don't overdo it, or it will get runny. When all else fails, add some sugar or natural sweeteners like honey, agave nectar, or stevia.

Do's and Don'ts of Safety with Your Machine Troubleshooting

Do's

- DO use cheetah spotted bananas
- DO use frozen fruit
- DO have ingredients measured and laid out
- DO experiment
- DO alternate the adding of ingredients

- DO thoroughly clean after every use

Don'ts

- **DO NOT** use ice
- **DO NOT** use fruits with pits
- **DO NOT** submerge the base of the machine in water
- **DO NOT** use a lot of liquid
- **DO NOT** use gummy candies
- **DO NOT** use hard candies

Troubleshooting

- What is my Yonanas Healthy Dessert Maker® turns off while I'm using it?

Make sure the chute is locked at the 12 o'clock position and has not slipped out. Sometimes if the machine runs for more than 3 minutes or gets hot, it will shut off. If all is as it should be, let the machine rest for 5 minutes and try again.

- What if I can't get my machine to turn on?

Make sure the unit is plugged in and the chute is locked at the 12 o'clock position. You should hear and feel the chute click into place when assembling the machine.

- What is it smells like it's burning?

There could be residue on the motor.

- What if nothing comes out after I put fruit in?

Make sure you are using enough fruit to push everything through the machine.

CHAPTER 7:

Cakes and Pies

1.   Lime Cake

Preparation Time: 5 Hours

Cooking Time: 0 Minutes **Servings:** 9

Ingredients:

- 15 Gingersnap cookies, crushed
- 1 ½ Cups almonds, crushed
- 1/3 Cup melted butter
- 2 Pints vanilla ice cream
- 2 Pints lime sorbet
- Whipped topping

Directions:

Combine the crushed cookies, crushed almonds, and butter in a bowl.

Next, press the mixture into a pie pan to form a crust.

Freeze for 15 minutes.

Feast the vanilla ice cream on top of the crust.

Cover with foil.

Next, freeze for 30 minutes.

Spread the sorbet on top.

Cover and freeze for 4 hours.

Lastly, top with the whipped topping before serving.

Nutrition: Calories: 174 Fat: 14g Saturated fat: 4.9g Carbohydrates: 9.4g Fiber: 2g Protein: 3.4g Cholesterol: 18mg Sugars: 5.6g Sodium: 51mg Potassium: 118mg

2. Banana Split Pie

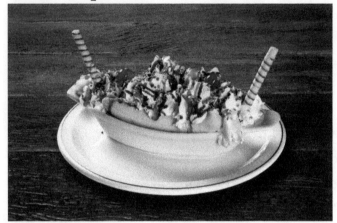

Preparation Time: 4 Hours and 15 Minutes

Cooking Time: 0 Minutes

Servings: 8

Ingredients:

- ½ Teaspoon lemon juice
- 3 Tablespoons of chocolate ice cream topping
- 1 Graham cracker crust
- 2 Bananas, sliced
- 8 Maraschino cherries
- 1 qt. Strawberry ice cream softened
- ½ Cup pineapple ice cream topping
- ½ Cup walnuts, chopped and toasted
- 2 cups whipped topping
- Chocolate syrup

Directions:

Place the crust in a pie pan.

Add the chocolate ice cream topping on top of the crust.

Freeze for 5 minutes.

Toss the bananas in lemon juice.

Sprinkle the bananas on top of the chocolate ice cream topping.

Add the pineapple ice cream topping, walnuts, strawberry ice cream, and whipped topping on top of the pie.

Cover the pie.

Freeze for 4 hours.

Drizzle with the chocolate syrup.

Garnish with the cherries before serving.

Nutrition:

- Calories: 459 Fat: 22g Saturated fat: 9g
- Carbohydrates: 64g Fiber: 2g
- Protein: 5g Cholesterol: 19mg Sugars: 26g
- Sodium: 174mg Potassium: 225mg

3.   Frozen Strawberry Lemonade Pie

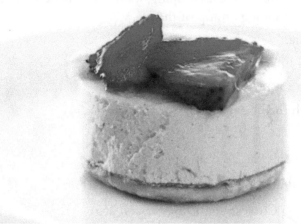

Preparation Time: 8 Hours and 20 Minutes

Cooking Time: 0 Minutes

Servings: 8

Ingredients:

- 2 ½ Cups strawberries, sliced
- 3 ½ oz. Lemon pudding mix
- 8 oz. Whipped topping
- 1 Graham cracker crust

Directions:

Combine the pudding mix and strawberries in a bowl.

Next, let sit for 5 minutes.

Stir in the whipped topping.

Then, add the graham cracker crust to a pie pan.

Top the crust with the strawberry mixture.

Freeze for 8 hours.

Nutrition:

- Calories: 306 Fat: 10g Saturated fat: 6g Carbohydrates: 51g
- Fiber: 2g Protein: 1g Cholesterol: 0mg
- Sugars: 45g Sodium: 273mg Potassium: 351mg

4. Chocolate & Hazelnut Caramel Pie

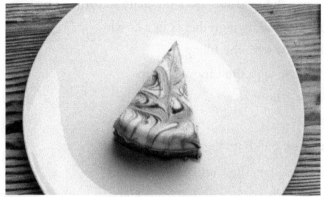

Preparation Time: 1 Hour and 40 Minutes

Cooking Time: 0 Minutes

Servings: 8

Ingredients:

- 12 Shortbread cookies, crushed
- 1 ½ Cups caramel pretzels, crushed
- ¼ Cup sugar
- 6 Tablespoons melted butter
- 3 Tablespoons caramel syrup

Filling

- ½ Cup chocolate hazelnut spread
- 8 oz. Cream cheese
- 7 oz. Marshmallow cream
- 8 oz. Whipped topping
- 2 oz. Chocolate bar, chopped
- 1 Cup marshmallows

Directions:

Add the cookies and pretzels to a food processor.

Next, pulse until crumbly.

Stir in the butter and sugar.

Process until fully combined.

Next, press the mixture into a pie plate to form a crust.

Combine the filling ingredients in a bowl.

Top the crust with the filling.

Then, drizzle with the caramel syrup.

Freeze for 1 hour.

Nutrition:

- Calories: 663 Fat: 35g
- Saturated fat: 19g Carbohydrates: 74g
- Fiber: 1g Protein: 6g Cholesterol: 60mg
- Sugars: 57g Sodium: 327mg Potassium: 445mg

5.   Caramel & Almond Ice Cream Cake

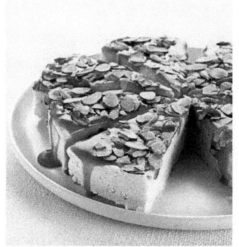

Preparation Time: 5 Hours and 20 Minutes

Cooking Time: 0 Minutes

Servings: 16

Ingredients:

- ¼ Cup melted butter
- 30 Pecan shortbread cookies, crushed
- 6 Cups butter pecan ice cream
- 8 oz. Whipped topping
- ¾ Cup toffee bits
- ¾ Cup almonds, slivered and toasted
- ¼ Cup caramel syrup

Directions:

Mix the butter and crushed cookies.

Next, press the mixture into a pie pan to form a crust.

Spread half of the butter pecan ice cream on top of the crust.

Freeze for 30 minutes.

Next, add more layers and freeze for 30 minutes.

For the topping, add the whipped topping and sprinkle with toffee bits and almonds.

Freeze for 4 hours.

Drizzle with the caramel syrup and serve.

Nutrition:

- Calories: 410
- Fat: 28g
- Saturated fat: 11g
- Carbohydrates: 36g
- Fiber: 1g
- Protein: 5g
- Cholesterol: 37mg
- Sugars: 19g
- Sodium: 232mg
- Potassium: 335mg

6.   Lemon Meringue Ice Cream Pie

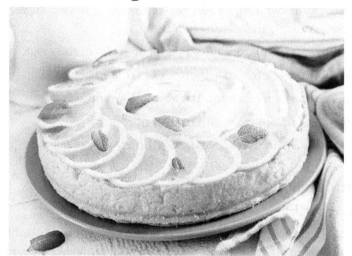

Preparation Time: 5 Hours and 30 Minutes

Cooking Time: 0 Minutes

Servings: 8

Ingredients:

Crust

- ¼ Cup melted butter
- ¼ Cup brown sugar
- 1 Cup graham cracker crumbs
- ¾ Cup pecans, chopped

Filling

- 1 qt. Vanilla ice cream, softened and divided
- 2 Tablespoons lemon juice
- 10 oz. Lemon curd

Meringue

- ¼ Teaspoon cream of tartar
- 6 Tablespoons sugar
- 4 Egg whites

Directions:

Preheat your oven to 400 degrees F. Add the butter, sugar, graham cracker crumbs, and pecans in a bowl.

Next, press the mixture into a pie plate to form the crust.

Bake in the oven for 10 minutes. Let cool on a wire rack.

Transfer to the freezer and freeze for 30 minutes.

Spread half of the ice cream on top of the crust.

Freeze for 30 minutes. Next, in a bowl, mix the lemon juice and lemon curd.

Spread this mixture on top of the ice cream.

Freeze for 1 hour. Add the remaining ice cream on top.

Freeze for another 2 hours. In a pan over medium heat, blend the sugar, cream of tartar, and egg whites. Then, using a hand mixer, beat the mixture on a low-speed setting for 1 minute.

Beat on medium speed until you see peaks forming.

Spread the meringue on top of the pie. Use a kitchen torch to broil the meringue for 3 minutes.

Freeze for 1 hour and serve.

Nutrition:

- Calories: 499 Fat: 24g Saturated fat: 10g Carbohydrates: 66g Fiber: 1g Protein: 6g
- Cholesterol: 71mg Sugars: 54g Sodium: 211mg Potassium: 343mg

CHAPTER 8:

Popsicles

7.   The British Pop

Preparation Time: 12 Hours and 6 Minutes

Cooking Time: 5 Hours

Servings: 6

Ingredients:

- 1 (12 oz.) cans evaporated milk
- 1 C. Heavy cream
- 4 Earl Grey teabags
- Finely chopped pistachios
- 1/2 Tsp ground cardamom
- 1 (14 oz.) cans sweetened condensed milk
- Chopped nuts for topping.

Directions:

Begin to heat your milk in a small pot until bubbles begin to show around the edges.

At the same time, remove the top part of your tea bags and combine the tea with the milk.

Add in the cardamom with the milk.

At this point, the milk should be gently boiling; shut off the heat, place a lid on the pot, then let the milk sit for 35 mins.

Now run the milk through a strainer into a bowl, then add in the condensed milk, pistachios, and cream.

Divide this mix between the popsicle molds and cover the molds with some plastic wrap.

Place everything in the freezer and let the mix sit in the freezer for 8 hours.

Place the mold under some warm water before serving the popsicles.

Top your popsicles with some nuts.

Enjoy.

Nutrition:

- Calories: 425.7 Fat: 24.7g Cholesterol: 93.2mg Sodium: 159.2mg
- Carbohydrates: 42.9g Protein: 9.9g

8.   The Countryside Pop
Preparation Time: 10 Minutes

Cooking Time: 30 Minutes

Servings: 3

Ingredients:

- 3 Bananas
- 1 Tbsp milk
- 6 oz. half a bag of chocolate chips
- 1 Tbsp icing sugar
- 1 Pinch nutmeg
- 1 Ash cinnamon

Directions:

Remove the skins of your bananas, then place them to the side.

Add your chips and the milk into a small pot and heat the chips until they are evenly melted.

Combine in the cinnamon and nutmeg and shut the heat.

Get a plate and line it with some parchment paper, then layer your bananas on top of the parchment paper.

Top the bananas with chocolate and try to cover the fruits nicely.

Now freeze everything for 40 mins.

Top your frozen bananas with some icing sugar and insert a stick into each one.

Enjoy.

Nutrition:

- Calories: 376.9
- Fat: 17.4g
- Cholesterol: 0.0mg
- Sodium: 7.4mg
- Carbohydrates: 62.7g Protein: 3.6g

9. The Latin Pop

Preparation Time: 15 Minutes

Cooking Time: 0 Minutes

Servings: 8

Ingredients:

- 1 C. water
- 1 Pinch salt
- 1/2 C. sugar
- 2 Tbsps. freshly squeezed lime juice
- 2 Small ripe avocados

Directions:

Add your sugar and water to a small pot, then begin to heat and stir the mix until everything is boiling.

Once the sugar is completely combined, shut the heat and let the mix get to room temp.

Now slice your avocados into two pieces, then take out the pit and remove the flesh into a food processor.

Add in the room temp mix, syrup, and some salt.

Pulse the mix until it is combined nicely, then add in the lime juice.

Separate your avocado mix between ice pop molds, then seal them with the lids and place everything in the freezer for 6 hrs.

Enjoy.

Nutrition:

- Calories: 121.6
- Fat: 6.6g
- Cholesterol: 0.0mg
- Sodium: 23.6mg
- Carbohydrates: 16.6g
- Protein: 0.9g

10.   The Sweety Pie Pop

Preparation Time: 4 Hours

Cooking Time: 0 Minutes

Servings: 1

Ingredients:

- 32 oz. Yogurt
- 1 Tbsp. approximately lemon juice
- 2 Bananas
- 15 oz. Mandarin oranges, drained, chopped
- 1/4 C. Chopped maraschino cherry
- 1/2 C. Sugar
- 1/2 C. roughly crushed pineapple in juice, undrained

Directions:

Add your bananas, then pulse them until they are pureed nicely.

Add the bananas to a bowl and add in the rest of the ingredients.

Stir the mix to combine everything nicely, then carefully divide the mix between ice pop molds.

Place your pops in the freezer for 60 mins.

Now stake your sticks into the molds and continue to freeze them until they are solid.

Enjoy.

Nutrition:

- Calories: 91.1
- Fat: 2.0g
- Cholesterol: 7.4mg
- Sodium: 27.1mg
- Carbohydrates: 17.1g
- Protein: 2.3g

11. The Orange and Green Machine Pop

Preparation Time: 20 Minutes

Cooking Time: 0 Minutes

Servings: 6

Ingredients:

- 1 C. Strawberry, hulled
- 1 1/2 C. Orange juice
- 2 Large kiwi fruits, peeled
- 1/2 C. Raspberries

Directions:

Cut your kiwi and strawberries into 12 pieces and divide the pieces between 6 cups.

Slice the remaining fruit and divide them between the cup. as well evenly.

Now divide your orange juice between the cup. And fill them, and put everything in the freezer.

After 65 mins of freezing time, stake a stick into each cup. And continue to freeze everything for four more hours.

At serving time, run the cup under some warm water and remove the popsicle.

Enjoy.

Nutrition:

- Calories: 59.4
- Fat: 0.4g
- Cholesterol: 0.0mg
- Sodium: 1.8mg
- Carbohydrates: 13.9g
- Protein: 1.0g

12. The Pink Pop

Preparation Time: 15 Minutes

Cooking Time: 2 Minutes

Servings: 1

Ingredients:

- 1 Tbsp. gelatin
- 1 Tbsp. fresh lemon juice or 1 tbsp lime juice 1/4 C. boiling water
- 1/2 seedless watermelon
- 1/2 C. granulated sugar

Directions:

Add your boiling water to a bowl and add your gelatin on top of the water.

Let the mix sit for 65 secs.

With a scooper, take out the flesh of your watermelon and divide the insides of the fruit between 4 cups.

Add your melon, lemon juice, and sugar to a blender and pulse the mix a few times.

Combine the melon mix with your gelatin mix and stir everything again, then divide the mix between ice pop molds and place the sticks into the molds immediately.

Place everything in the freezer for at least 4 hours.

Enjoy.

Nutrition:

- Calories: 68.2
- Fat: 0.2g
- Cholesterol: 0.0mg
- Sodium: 2.4mg
- Carbohydrates: 16.9g
- Protein: 1.2g

13.   The Brown and Pink Pop

Preparation Time: 30 Minutes

Cooking Time: 0 Minutes

Servings: 24

Ingredients:

- 1 Small watermelon, seedless
- 2 pt. Lime sherbet softened
- 1 C. sugar
- 1/2 C. mini chocolate chips

Directions:

Remove the flesh of your watermelon and divide it between 10 cups.

Add the melon to a blender and also add in the sugar; working in batches, pulse the mix into an even puree.

Now run the mix through a strainer into a bowl, then place a covering on the bowl and put everything in the freezer for about 3 hours until it is partly frozen.

Add in the chocolate pieces.

Divide the mix between 24 plastic cups. Evenly, leaving about 1 inch of space, then put everything back in the freezer for three more hours.

Divide your sherbet over each cup. Evenly, and place a covering of plastic over each one.

Cut an opening into the covering and stake a stick into each cup, carefully.

Push the stick in as far as possible to increase its strength.

Place everything back in the freezer overnight for up to 48 hours.

Enjoy.

Nutrition: Calories: 135.9 Fat: 1.8g Cholesterol: 0.2mg Sodium: 13.5mg Carbohydrates: 30.9g Protein: 1.4g

14. The United States of Pop

Preparation Time: 5 Minutes

Cooking Time: 0 Minutes

Servings: 6

Ingredients:

- 3 C. vanilla yogurt
- Wax paper
- Red food coloring
- 6 Sugar ice cream cones
- White food coloring
- 6 Wooden popsicle sticks
- Blue food coloring

Directions:

Add some red food coloring to half a 1/2 cup. of yogurt and color 1.5 cups of yogurt with blue food coloring.

Keep the remaining yogurt white.

Layout 6 pieces of wax paper that are about 1 foot in size.

Fold them into triangles.

Use each triangle as a covering for your sugar cones and tape them to the cone to preserve the structure.

Add 1 tablespoon of red yogurt, 2 tablespoons of white, and 3 tablespoons of blue.

Add in your stick and place everything in the freezer for 5 hrs.

Enjoy.

Nutrition:

- Calories: 114.9
- Fat: 4.3g
- Cholesterol: 15.9mg
- Sodium: 88.3mg
- Carbohydrates: 14.1g Protein: 5.0gr

15.   The Sophia Pop

Preparation Time: 5 Minutes

Cooking Time: 0 Minutes

Servings: 4

Ingredients:

- 1 C. plain yogurt
- 4 Paper C. 5 oz. size
- 1 C. fresh fruit
- Aluminum foil
- 2 Tbsps. honey
- 4 Wooden popsicle sticks

Directions:

Add the following to a food processor: honey, fruit, and yogurt. Pulse the mix until it is smooth, then divide the mix between the cup. Leaving about 1/4 of space in each cup.

Place a covering on each cut and slice a little opening into each one.

Stake your sticks into each cup carefully, then put everything in the fridge for 6 hours.

Enjoy.

Nutrition:

- Calories: 69.2
- Fat: 1.9g
- Cholesterol: 7.9mg
- Sodium: 28.6mg
- Carbohydrates: 11.5g
- Protein: 2.1g

16.   Spiced Apple Cider Sorbet

Preparation Time: 5 Minutes

Cooking Time: 5 Minutes

Servings: 2 to 4

Ingredients:

- 6 Frozen apples, peeled, cored, and seeded
- 3 Tablespoons fresh-pressed apple juice
- 1 Teaspoon honey
- 1 Teaspoon grated cloves
- 2 Teaspoons cinnamon
- 1/2 Teaspoon fresh lemon juice
- 2 Tablespoons spiced rum

Directions:

Place a large mixing bowl under the fruit chute and push the apples through.

Add apple juice, honey, clove, cinnamon, lemon juice, and spiced rum to the mixing bowl.

Mix until smooth to blend the flavors.

Spoon into individual bowls.

Freeze leftovers in an airtight container.

Nutrition:

- Calories: 174
- Sodium: 4mg
- Dietary Fiber: 7.4g
- Total Fat: 0.6g
- Total Carbs: 41.8g
- Protein: 0.8g

17.   Concord Grape Sorbet

Preparation Time: 3 Minutes

Cooking Time: 5 Minutes

Servings: 2 to 3

Ingredients:

- 4 Cups frozen Concord grapes, stemmed

Directions:

Place a large mixing bowl under the fruit chute and push the grapes through.

Spoon into individual bowls.

Freeze leftovers in an airtight container.

Nutrition:

- Calories: 62

- Sodium: 2mg

- Dietary Fiber: 0.8g

- Total Fat: 0.3g

- Total Carbs: 15.8g

- Protein: 0.6g

18.   Homemade Coco-Mango Sorbet

Preparation Time: 5 Minutes

Cooking Time: 5 Minutes

Servings: 3

Ingredients:

- 3 Frozen mangoes, chopped
- 3 Tablespoons unsweetened coconut milk
- 1/2 Cup coconut cream, chilled
- 1 Teaspoon pure vanilla extract
- 1 Teaspoon honey
- 1/4 Cup unsweetened coconut, shredded

Directions:

Place a large mixing bowl under the fruit chute and push the mangos through.

Add coconut milk, coconut cream, vanilla extract, and honey; mix until well-blended.

Scoop into separate bowls and top with shredded coconut.

Freeze leftovers in an airtight container.

Nutrition:

- Calories: 231
- Sodium: 12mg
- Dietary Fiber: 3.6g
- Total Fat: 15.6g
- Total Carbs: 23.2g
- Protein: 2.0g

19.   Citrus-Mint Sorbet

Preparation Time: 5 Minutes

Cooking Time: 25 Minutes

Servings: 5

Ingredients:

- 3 Frozen bananas
- 6 Frozen lemons, peeled and seeded
- 3 Frozen oranges, peeled and seeded
- 1 Cup Greek yogurt
- 1 Tablespoon honey
- 2 Tablespoons fresh mint, chopped

Directions:

Place a large mixing bowl under the fruit chute and push the bananas, lemons, and oranges through.

Mix in yogurt and honey until well-blended.

Fold in chopped mint.

Spoon into individual bowls, and freeze leftover soft-serve in an airtight container.

Nutrition:

- Calories: 184
- Sodium: 18mg
- Dietary Fiber: 6.6g
- Total Fat: 1.5g
- Total Carbs: 41.1g
- Protein: 7.3g

20. Lemon-Aid Sorbet

Preparation Time: 5 Minutes

Cooking Time: 20 Minutes

Servings: 2 to 4

Ingredients:

- 2 Cups water
- 4 Black or orange pekoe tea bags
- 3 Frozen bananas, peeled
- 1/4 Cup lemon juice
- 1 Tablespoon bourbon
- 1 Teaspoon honey

Directions:

Bring two cups of water to a boil on high heat in a medium saucepan.

Add tea bags and remove from heat.

Steep the tea for 15 to 20 minutes.

Pour the tea into two ice cube trays and freeze overnight.

Place a mixing bowl under the fruit chute and push the bananas and tea ice cubes through.

Add lemon juice, bourbon, and honey to the mixing bowl.

Blend until smooth.

Spoon into individual bowls and freeze leftover soft-serve in an airtight container.

Nutrition:

- Calories: 96
- Sodium: 8mg
- Dietary Fiber: 2.4g
- Total Fat: 0.4g
- Total Carbs: 23.0g
- Protein: 1.1g

21.   Rosé Sherbet

Preparation Time: 5 Minutes

Cooking Time: 5 Minutes

Servings: 3 to 5

Ingredients:

- 3 Cups frozen raspberries
- 1/2 Cup rosé wine
- Rose petals for garnish

Directions:

Place a large mixing bowl under the fruit chute and push the raspberries through.

Add rosé wine and mix until well-blended

Scoop into champagne glasses and add a rose petal or two for garnish.

Nutrition:

- Calories: 58
- Sodium: 2mg
- Dietary Fiber: 4.8g
- Total Fat: 0.5g
- Total Carbs: 9.5g
- Protein: 0.9g

22.   Oat & Dulce de Leche Sorbet

Preparation Time: 5 Minutes

Cooking Time: 5 Minutes

Servings: 4 to 6

Ingredients:

- 9 Frozen bananas, peeled
- 1/2 Cup Greek yogurt, vanilla flavored
- 1 Teaspoon honey
- 1 Teaspoon spiced rum, frozen
- 1 Cup honey toasted granola
- 1/2 Cup dulce de leche

Directions:

Place a mixing bowl under the fruit chute and push the bananas through.

Add yogurt, honey, and spiced rum to the mixing bowl.

Blend until smooth.

Fold in the honey toasted granola.

Spoon into individual bowls, and drizzle with dulce de leche.

Nutrition:

- Calories: 304
- Sodium: 51mg
- Dietary Fiber: 8.3g
- Total Fat: 11.9g
- Total Carbs: 79.5g
- Protein: 12.1g

23. **Banana Sorbet with Rose and Pistachio**

Preparation Time: 5 Minutes

Cooking Time: 5 Minutes

Servings: 2 to 4

Ingredients:

- 6 Frozen bananas, peeled
- 1/4 Cup Greek yogurt, vanilla flavored
- 1 Tablespoon honey
- 1/2 Teaspoon rose water
- 1/2 Cup pistachios, chopped

Directions:

Place a mixing bowl under the fruit chute and push the bananas through.

Add yogurt, honey, and rose water to the mixing bowl.

Blend until smooth.

Spoon into individual bowls, and top each serving with a generous portion of chopped pistachios.

Freeze leftover soft-serve in an airtight container.

Nutrition:

- Calories: 224
- Sodium: 47mg
- Dietary Fiber: 5.4g
- Total Fat: 4.4g
- Total Carbs: 47.3g
- Protein: 4.9g

24. Lemon Drop Sorbet

Preparation Time: 5 Minutes

Cooking Time: 5 Minutes

Servings: 2

Ingredients:

- 4 Frozen bananas, peeled
- 4 Tablespoons fresh lemon juice, frozen
- 3 Tablespoons lemon zest
- 1 Teaspoon honey
- 1 Tablespoon vodka
- 1/2 Teaspoon pink Himalayan salt

Directions:

Place a large mixing bowl under the fruit chute.

Push the frozen bananas through the chute.

Add frozen lemon juice, zest, honey, vodka, and salt to the mixing bowl.

Mix until well-blended.

Spoon into individual bowls.

Freeze leftovers in an airtight container.

Nutrition:

- Calories: 250
- Sodium: 590mg
- Dietary Fiber: 6.8g
- Total Fat: 1.1g
- Total Carbs: 59.3g
- Protein: 3.0g

25.   Mango Tango Sorbet

Preparation Time: 5 Minutes

Cooking Time: 5 Minutes

Servings: 4

Ingredients:

- 1 Bag frozen mango
- 1 Frozen orange, peeled and seeded
- 5 Frozen tangerines, peeled and seeded
- 3 Tablespoons lime juice
- 1 Tablespoon lime zest

Directions:

Place a large mixing bowl under the fruit chute.

Push the frozen mango, orange, and tangerines through the fruit chute.

Add the lime juice, then zest to the mixing bowl.

Mix until well-blended.

Spoon into discrete bowls, and freeze leftovers in an airtight container.

Nutrition:

- Calories: 121
- Sodium: 8mg
- Dietary Fiber: 3.4g
- Total Fat: 0.3g
- Total Carbs: 31.0g
- Protein: 1.7g

CHAPTER 9:

Alcoholic Treats

26.   Coffee Rum Ice Cream

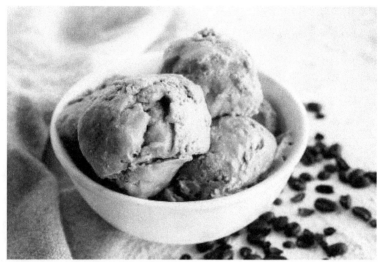

Preparation Time: 3 to 4 Hours

Cooking Time: 0 Minutes

Servings: 4

Ingredients:

- 4 oz. Dark rum
- 8 Scoops vanilla ice cream
- 4 Cups brewed coffee, at room temperature
- 1/4 Cup semisweet chocolate chips, melted
- 1/2 Cup coffee-flavored liqueur

Directions:

Combine 1/2 cup coffee-flavored liqueur to a measuring cup along with 4 cups brewed coffee and dark rum.

Mix the vanilla ice cream with the rum coffee mixture, transfer the ice cream mixture to a container, and freeze for 40 minutes. After 40 minutes, remove it from the freezer and stir very well with a fork or a spatula.

Freeze for another 40 minutes. Top with melted chocolate and enjoy!

Nutrition:

- Calories: 148
- Fat: 22g
- Total carbs: 3g
- Protein: 2g

27.   **Prosecco Ice Cream**

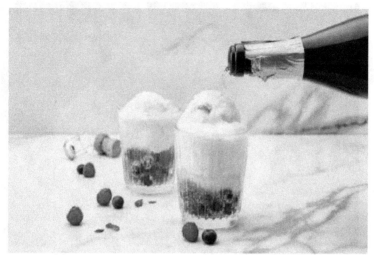

Preparation Time: 4 to 5 Hours

Cooking Time: 0 Minutes

Servings: 4

Ingredients:

- 2 Tablespoons honey
- 2 Tablespoons Prosecco
- 2 Cups heavy cream
- 1 Can condensed milk, sweetened

Directions:

Beat heavy cream in a stand mixer for about 5 minutes, until stiff peaks form.

Fold in 2 tablespoons of honey and sweetened condensed milk, process until combined well. Then add in 2 tablespoons Prosecco.

Transfer this mixture to a loaf pan. Freeze for 4 to 5 hours.

Just before serving, let it soften for 10 minutes, then serve and enjoy.

Nutrition: Calorie: 306 Fat: 25.8g Total carbs: 16g Protein: 5g

28. Margarita Pops

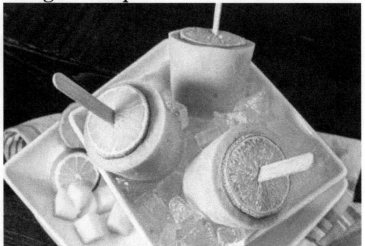

Preparation Time: 5 to 6 Hours

Cooking Time: 0 Minutes

Servings: 4

Ingredients:

- 1 Tablespoon orange liqueur
- 1/2 Cup fresh lime juice
- 1/2 Can condensed milk, sweetened
- 2 Limes, sliced
- 1/2 Cup of water
- 1 Cup fresh or frozen strawberries
- 1/8 Cup Tequila
- 1 Cup of frozen mango

Directions:

Add fresh lime juice, tequila, sweetened condensed milk, orange liqueur, and water to a large bowl. Stir well.

Take 2 Dixie cups and divide 1/3 of the mixture among them.

Transfer 1/3 of the combination to a blender along with the mango. Add more water, if needed, and blend until creamy and smooth. Once done, divide among two other Dixie cups.

Rinse the blender and transfer the leftover base to a blender. Add in fresh or frozen strawberries and more water, if needed. Blend until smooth and equally divide among the remaining Dixie cups.

Take lime slices and insert popsicle sticks into each slice. Top each cup with lime slices. There should be no room between the lime slice and the ice cream mixture. Freeze overnight or for at least 5 hours.

Just before serving, open the Dixie cups with scissors and remove them from the pops.

Serve and enjoy!

Nutrition:

- Calories: 128
- Fat: 3.8g
- Total carbs: 22g
- Protein: 4g

29. Mudslide Ice Cream

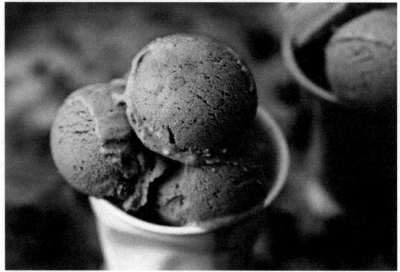

Preparation Time: 3 to 4 Hours

Cooking Time: 15 Minutes

Servings: 4

Ingredients:

- 1 Cup chocolate, chopped
- 2 Tablespoons Baileys Irish Cream
- 2 Cups heavy cream
- 2 Tablespoons Kahlua
- 1 Can (14.5-oz.) sweetened condensed milk
- 1/4 Cup hot fudge sauce

Directions:

Beat heavy cream in a stand mixer for about 5 minutes, until stiff peaks form.

Fold in the sweetened condensed milk, then stir well until combined. Then fold in 2 tablespoons Kahlua, 1 cup chopped chocolate, 1/4 cup hot fudge sauce, and two tablespoons Baileys Irish Cream.

Transfer this mixture to a loaf pan and top with more chocolate. Freeze for about 4 to 5 hours.

Just before serving, let it soften for 10 minutes.

Serve and enjoy!

Nutrition:

- Calories: 525
- Fat: 29.4g
- Total carbs: 58g
- Protein: 7g

30.   Coffee Vodka Ice Cream

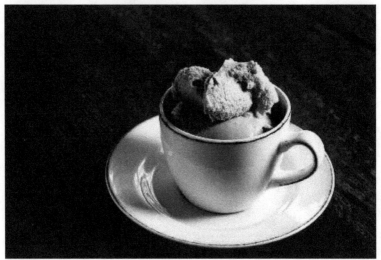

Preparation Time: 3 to 4 Hours

Cooking Time: 10 Minutes

Servings: 4

Ingredients:

- 2 Tablespoons instant coffee
- 1/2 Cup vodka
- 1.5 Cups water, hot
- 3 Cups coconut cream
- 1.5 Cups sugar
- 2 Cups whipped cream, beaten until stiff peaks form
- 1 Tablespoon vanilla extract

Directions:

Pour hot water into the coffee and mix to combine. Preheat a pan over medium heat.

Add coconut cream, coffee, and sugar. You may also add a pinch of salt.

Cook for about 5 minutes, stirring constantly.

Remove from heat and add vodka, cream, and vanilla; stir well to combine.

Handover the ice cream mixture to a container and freeze for 40 minutes; after 40 minutes, remove it from the freezer and stir very well with a fork or a spatula.

Freeze for another 40 minutes. Repeat the procedure 3-4 more times or until the ice cream is frozen.

Serve and enjoy!

Nutrition:

- Calories: 365
- Fat: 16.6g
- Total carbs: 48g
- Protein: 7g

CHAPTER 10:

Sorbet

31.   Mojito Sorbet

Preparation Time: 5 Minutes

Cooking Time: 5 Minutes

Servings: 4

Ingredients:

- 6 Frozen bananas, peeled
- 5 Sprigs of mint, chopped
- 3 Tablespoons freshly-squeezed lime juice
- 3 Tablespoons dark rum, frozen
- 1 Teaspoon lime zest

Directions:

Place a large mixing bowl under the fruit chute.

Push frozen bananas through the chute.

Add mint, lime juice, frozen rum, and zest to the mixing bowl.

Mix until smooth.

Spoon into individual bowls.

Freeze leftovers in an airtight container.

Nutrition:

- Calories: 193
- Sodium: 7mg
- Dietary Fiber: 5.7g
- Total Fat: 0.7g
- Total Carbs: 43.5gProtein: 2.5g

32.   Lime-Basil Sorbet

Preparation Time: 5 Minutes

Cooking Time: 5 Minutes

Servings: 4

Ingredients:

- 6 Frozen bananas, peeled
- 1/2 Cup freshly-squeezed lime juice
- 2 Tablespoons lime zest
- 3 Tablespoons fresh basil, chopped
- A sprig of fresh basil to garnish for parties

Directions:

Place a large mixing bowl under the fruit chute.

Push the frozen bananas through the chute.

Add lime juice, zest, and basil to the mixing bowl.

Mix until well-blended.

Spoon into individual bowls.

Freeze leftovers in an airtight container.

Nutrition:

- Calories: 161
- Sodium: 2mg
- Dietary Fiber: 5.0g
- Total Fat: 0.6g
- Total Carbs: 41.4g
- Protein: 2.1g

33. Zucchini-Lemon Sorbet

Preparation Time: 5 Minutes

Cooking Time: 5 Minutes

Servings: 4

Ingredients:

- 3 Frozen bananas, peeled
- 2 Frozen zucchinis, peeled
- 1/4 Cup lemon juice
- 1 Tablespoon lemon zest

Directions:

Place a large mixing bowl under the fruit chute.

Push the frozen bananas through the chute.

Push the zucchini through the chute.

Add the lemon juice, then zest to the mixing bowl.

Mix until well-blended.

Spoon into separate bowls, and freeze leftovers in an airtight container.

Nutrition:

- Calories: 99
- Sodium: 14mg
- Dietary Fiber: 3.5g
- Total Fat: 0.6g
- Total Carbs: 24.1g
- Protein: 2.3g

34. Raspberry-Campari Sorbet

Preparation Time: 5 Minutes

Cooking Time: 5 Minutes

Servings: 2 to 4

Ingredients:

- 5 Cups frozen raspberries
- 2 Tablespoons honey
- 3 Tablespoons Campari
- 1 Teaspoon fresh-squeezed orange juice
- 1/2 Teaspoon fresh orange zest
- 1/4 Teaspoon kosher salt
- 1/2 Teaspoon fresh lemon juice

Directions:

Place a large mixing bowl under the fruit chute.

Push the frozen raspberries through the chute.

Add honey, Campari, orange juice & zest, lemon juice, and salt to the mixing bowl.

Mix until well-blended.

Spoon into individual bowls.

Freeze leftovers in an airtight container.

Nutrition:

- Calories: 192.3
- Sodium: 197mg
- Dietary Fiber: 13.4g
- Total Fat: 1.3g
- Total Carbs: 40.5g
- Protein: 2.5g

35.   Pink Grapefruit Sorbet

Preparation Time: 15 Minutes

Cooking Time: 3 Minutes

Servings: 2

Ingredients:

- 6 Frozen grapefruits, peeled

Directions:

Prep the grapefruit by cutting each in half; peel and deseed. Make sure all of the rind (hard skin) is separated from the fruit.

Freeze all of the fruit in an airtight container overnight.

When you're ready to make the soft-serve, place a large mixing bowl under the fruit chute.

Push the frozen grapefruit spears through the chute using the plunger.

Mix the soft-serve together until smooth.

Spoon into separate bowls, and freeze leftovers in an airtight container.

Nutrition:

- Calories: 123
- Sodium: 0mg
- Dietary Fiber: 4.2g
- Total Fat: 0.4g
- Total Carbs: 31.0g
- Protein: 2.4g

36.   Apple Sorbet

Preparation Time: 5 Minutes

Cooking Time: 5 Minutes

Servings: 3 to 5

Ingredients:

- 5 Frozen apples, peeled, cored, and deseeded
- 3 Tablespoons fresh-pressed apple juice
- 1/2 Teaspoon lemon juice

Directions:

Place a large mixing bowl under the fruit chute and push the apples through.

Add apple and lemon juice.

Stir until smooth.

Spoon into separate bowls and freeze leftovers in an airtight container.

Nutrition:

- Calories: 165
- Sodium: 3mg
- Dietary Fiber: 7.4g
- Total Fat: 0.6g
- Total Carbs: 43.7g
- Protein: 0.8g

37.   Pineapple Sorbet

Preparation Time: 5 Minutes

Cooking Time: 3 to 5 Minutes

Servings: 2

Ingredients:

- 1 Small bag of frozen pineapple chunks or one small pineapple, peeled, cored, and frozen

Directions:

Put frozen bananas through the chute. Using the plunger, push the pineapple down the chute.

Push frozen pineapple through the chute.

Mix the soft-serve together until smooth.

Spoon into individual bowls.

Nutrition:

- Calories: 41
- Sodium: 1mg
- Dietary Fiber: 1.1g
- Total Fat: 0.1g
- Total Carbs: 10.8g
- Protein: 0.4g

38. Raspberry and Redcurrant Sorbet

Preparation Time: 5 Minutes

Cooking Time: 5 Minutes

Servings: 2 to 4

Ingredients:

- 5 Cups frozen raspberries
- 2 Cups frozen redcurrants, destemmed

Directions:

Place a large mixing bowl under the fruit chute and push the raspberries and redcurrants through.

Stir until smooth to blend the flavors.

Spoon into separate bowls and freeze leftovers in an airtight container.

Nutrition:

- Calories: 160
- Sodium: 3mg
- Dietary Fiber: 20.0g
- Total Fat: 2.0g
- Total Carbs: 36.7g
- Protein: 3.7g

39. Red Plum Sorbet

Preparation Time: 5 Minutes

Cooking Time: 5 Minutes

Servings: 2 to 4

Ingredients:

- 9 Frozen plums, pitted and quartered
- 1/3 Teaspoon cardamom powder
- 3 Tablespoons of honey
- 1 Teaspoon lemon juice

Directions:

Place a large mixing bowl under the fruit chute and push the plums through.

Add cardamom powder, honey, and lemon juice to the mixing bowl.

Mix until smooth to blend the flavors.

Spoon into individual bowls.

Freeze leftovers in an airtight container.

Nutrition:

- Calories: 93
- Sodium: 1mg
- Dietary Fiber: 1.4g
- Total Fat: 0.3g
- Total Carbs: 24.3g
- Protein: 0.8g

CHAPTER 11:

Banana Free Ice Cream

40.   Peach Ice Cream

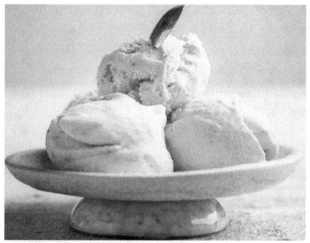

Preparation Time: 25 Minutes

Cooking Time: 0 Minutes

Servings: 8

Ingredients:

- 1-pound Fresh peaches, diced into small cubes
- ¾ Cup fine sugar
- 5 Egg yolks
- 1 ½ Cup heavy cream
- 1 Teaspoon vanilla extract

Directions:

Freeze the ice cream maker bowl rendering to manufacturer instructions, typically 12 to 24 hours.

Meanwhile, in a large saucepan, add the cream over medium-low heat. Bring the mixture to a soft simmer for about 10 to 12 minutes. Set aside.

In a mixing bowl, add the sugar and the egg yolks and whisk to combine. While stirring constantly, pour in the hot cream mixture slowly to temper the egg yolks.

Pour the mixture back into the saucepan and heat the whole mixture again over medium-low heat until creamy and thickened. You know it's prepared when the combination coats the back of a spoon.

Pour the mixture in a clean bowl over a fine-mesh sieve to strain and remove any cooked pieces of the egg yolks.

In the strained mixture, pour in the vanilla extract and mix until everything is combined. Let cool at room temperature.

Cover the combination with plastic wrap and let the combination cool in the fridge for at least 2 to 12 hours.

Pull out the ice cream combination from the fridge and stir a few times.

Mount the frozen ice cream maker container and pour the mixture into the ice cream maker.

Fix the machine and press ice cream and the start button.

About 5 to 6 minutes before the end of the churning process, add the chopped peaches pieces little by little into the ice cream and let it mix in.

When the cycle is over, transfer the ice cream to an airtight freezer-safe container or serve right away. If you like a harder consistency, allow the ice cream to freeze for 2 hours or more before serving.

Nutrition:

- Calories: 381 Fat: 22g Carbs: 43g Sugar: 41g Protein: 5g Sodium: 27mg

41. Pistachio Ice Cream

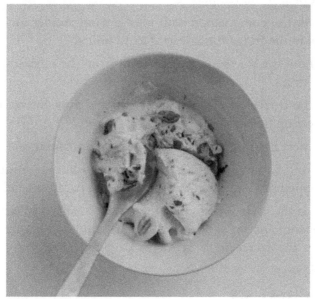

Preparation Time: 25 Minutes

Cooking Time: 0 Minutes

Servings: 8

Ingredients:

- 2 Cups heavy cream
- ¾ Cup honey
- 1 Teaspoon vanilla extract
- 1 Cup whole milk
- 1 Cup crushed pistachios

Directions:

Freeze the ice cream maker bowl rendering to manufacturer directions, usually 12 to 24 hours.

Meanwhile, in a large saucepan, add the cream, milk, and honey over medium-low heat. Bring the mixture to a soft simmer for about 10 to 12 minutes. Set aside.

Stir in the vanilla extract.

Pour the mixture into a clean bowl, preferably with a spout, and let it cool at room temperature.

Cover the combination with plastic wrap and let the combination cool in the fridge for at least 2 to 12 hours.

Pull out the ice cream combination from the refrigerator and stir a few times.

Fit the frozen ice cream maker bowl and pour the mixture into the ice cream maker.

Connect the machine, then press ice cream and the start button.

Around 5 minutes before the end of the churning process, add the chopped pistachios little by little into the ice cream and let it mix in.

When the cycle is over, transfer the ice cream to an airtight freezer-safe container or serve right away. If you like a harder consistency, allow the ice cream to freeze for 2 hours or more before serving.

Nutrition:

- Calories: 515
- Fat: 30g
- Carbs: 61g
- Sugar: 56g
- Protein: 7g
- Sodium: 137mg

42. Hazelnut Ice Cream

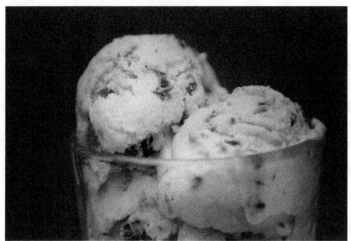

Preparation Time: 25 Minutes

Cooking Time: 0 Minutes

Servings: 8

Ingredients:

- 1 Cup whole milk
- ¾ Cup powdered sugar
- 2 Teaspoons vanilla extract
- 2 Cups crushed hazelnuts
- 2 Cups heavy cream

Directions:

Freeze the ice cream maker bowl rendering to manufacturer directions, usually 12 to 24 hours.

Meanwhile, in a large mixing bowl, add the cream, milk, and powdered sugar and whisk until completely incorporated.

Stir in the vanilla extract.

Cover the combination with plastic wrap and let the combination cool in the fridge for at least 2 to 12 hours.

Pull out the ice cream combination from the fridge and stir it a few times.

Mount the frozen ice cream maker bowl, then pour the mixture into it.

Attach the machine, then press ice cream and the start button.

About 5 to 6 minutes before the end of the churning process, add the crushed hazelnuts little by little into the ice cream and let it mix in.

When the cycle is ended, transfer the ice cream to an airtight freezer-safe container or serve right away. If you like a harder consistency, allow the ice cream to freeze for 2 hours or more before serving.

Nutrition:

- Calories: 573
- Fat: 47g
- Carbs: 33.4g
- Sugar: 27g
- Protein: 9g
- Sodium: 48mg

43.   Hazelnut and Chocolate Ice Cream

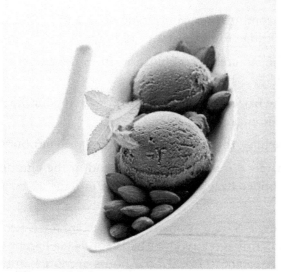

Preparation Time: 25 Minutes

Cooking Time: 0 Minutes

Servings: 8

Ingredients:

- 1 Cup whole milk
- 4 Tablespoons cocoa powder
- 2 Cups heavy cream
- ¾ Cup powdered sugar
- 2 Teaspoons vanilla extract
- 1 ½ cups crushed hazelnuts

Directions:

Freeze the ice cream maker bowl rendering to manufacturer instructions, typically 12 to 24 hours.

Meanwhile, in a large saucepan, add the cream, milk, cocoa powder, and powdered sugar over medium heat. Bring the mixture to a soft simmer for about 10 to 12 minutes. Set aside.

Stir in the vanilla extract.

Pour the mixture into a clean bowl and let it cool to room temperature.

Cover the combination with plastic wrap and let the combination cool in the fridge for at least 2 to 12 hours.

Pull out the ice cream combination from the fridge and whisk to mix it well.

Connect the frozen ice cream maker bowl and pour the mixture into the ice cream maker.

Fix the machine, then press ice cream and the start button.

Approximately 5 minutes before the end of the churning process, add the chopped hazelnuts little by little into the ice cream and let it mix in.

When the cycle is done, transfer the ice cream to an airtight freezer-safe container or serve right away. If you like a harder consistency, allow the ice cream to freeze for 2 hours or more before serving.

Nutrition:

- Calories: 526 Fat: 42g
- Carbs: 35g Sugar: 27g
- Protein: 8g Sodium: 49mg

44. Mango and Coconut Milk Ice Cream

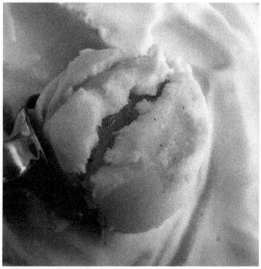

Preparation Time: 25 Minutes

Cooking Time: 0 Minutes

Servings: 8

Ingredients:

- 3 Cups mango, peeled and cut into cubes
- ¼ Cup whole milk
- ¾ Cup powdered sugar
- 1 ½ Cups heavy cream
- ½ Cup coconut milk

Directions:

Freeze the ice cream maker bowl rendering to manufacturer instructions, frequently 12 to 24 hours.

Meanwhile, in a large mixing bowl, add the milk, powdered sugar, heavy cream, and coconut milk.

Mix until everything is combined.

Cover the combination with plastic wrap and let the combination cool in the fridge for at least 2 to 12 hours.

Pull out the ice cream combination from the fridge and stir a few times.

Mount the frozen ice cream maker bowl and pour the mixture into it.

Join the machine and press ice cream and the start button.

About 5 to 6 minutes before the end of the churning process, add the diced mango pieces little by little into the ice cream and let it mix in.

When the cycle is done, transfer the ice cream to an airtight freezer-safe container or serve right away. If you like a harder consistency, allow the ice cream to freeze for 2 hours or more before serving.

Nutrition:

- Calories: 395
- Fat: 25g
- Carbs: 45g
- Sugar: 41g
- Protein: 3g
- Sodium: 29mg

45.   Avocado and Mint Ice Cream

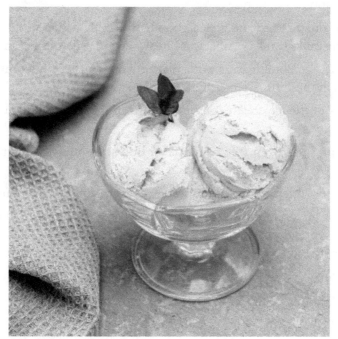

Preparation Time: 25 Minutes

Cooking Time: 0 Minutes

Servings: 8

Ingredients:

- 3 Avocados, peeled, cored, and diced
- 3 Tablespoons chopped mint
- ¾ Cup whole milk
- 2 Teaspoons vanilla extract
- ¾ Cup powdered sugar
- 1 ½ Cups heavy cream

Directions:

Freeze the ice cream maker bowl rendering to manufacturer instructions, typically 12 to 24 hours.

Meanwhile, in a high-speed blender, add the avocado, chopped mint, and powdered sugar.

Blitz until you achieved a smooth and creamy combination; it will take about 3 minutes.

Pour the mixture into a clean bowl, preferably with a spout, and stir in the milk, vanilla extract, and heavy cream. Mix until combined.

Cover the combination with plastic wrap and let the combination cool in the refrigerator for at least 2 to 12hours.

Pull out the ice cream combination from the fridge and stir it a few times.

Mount the frozen ice cream maker bowl and pour the mixture into it.

Connect the machine, then press ice cream and the start button.

When the cycle is over, transfer the ice cream to an airtight freezer-safe container or serve right away. If you like a harder consistency, allow the ice cream to freeze for 2 hours or more before serving.

Nutrition:

- Calories: 586
- Fat: 48g
- Carbs: 39g
- Sugar: 26g
- Protein: 5g
- Sodium: 46mg

46. Papaya and Passion Fruit Ice Cream

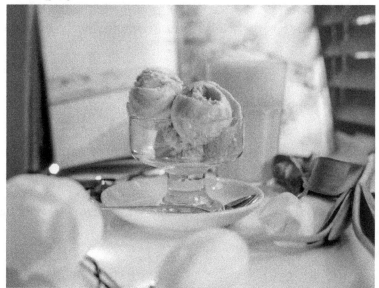

Preparation Time: 25 Minutes

Cooking Time: 0 Minutes

Servings: 8

Ingredients:

- 3 Cups papaya, peeled and diced into cubes
- ¾ Cup whole milk
- 3 Passion fruits, pulp out
- 1 Teaspoon vanilla extract
- ¾ Cup powdered sugar
- 2 Cups heavy cream

Directions:

Freeze the ice cream maker bowl rendering to manufacturer directions, usually 12 to 24 hours.

Meanwhile, in a high-speed blender, add the papaya, milk, passion fruit pulp, and powdered sugar.

Blitz until you get a smooth and combined mixture; it will take about 3 minutes.

Pour the mixture into a clean bowl, preferably with a spout, and stir in the vanilla extract and heavy cream. Mix until combined.

Cover the combination with plastic wrap and let the combination cool in the fridge for at least 2 to 12 hours.

Pull out the ice cream combination from the fridge and stir a few times.

Connect the frozen ice cream maker bowl and pour the mixture into it.

Attach the machine and press ice cream and the start button.

When the cycle is complete, transfer the ice cream to an airtight freezer-safe container or serve right away. If you like a harder consistency, allow the ice cream to freeze for 2 hours or more before serving.

Nutrition:

- Calories: 385
- Fat: 24g
- Carbs: 41g
- Sugar: 35g
- Protein: 4g
- Sodium: 54mg

47.   **Salted Caramel Ice Cream**

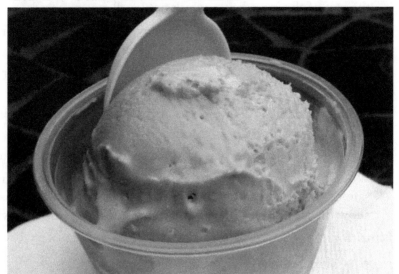

Preparation Time: 25 Minutes

Cooking Time: 0 Minutes

Servings: 8

Ingredients:

- 1 ¼ Cup sugar
- 1 Cup heavy cream
- ½ Teaspoon salt
- 1 Teaspoon vanilla extract
- 1 Cup whole milk
- 1 ½ Cup cream

Directions:

Freeze the ice cream maker bowl rendering to manufacturer instructions, typically 12 to 24 hours.

Meanwhile, in a saucepan, warm the sugar over medium heat until melted and amber color develops.

Stir in the heavy cream, then simmer for 5 minutes. Set aside.

Stir in the salt and let it cool completely.

In a mixing bowl, add the whole milk, pour caramel mixture, and the rest of the ingredients, whisk until well incorporated.

Cover the combination with plastic wrap and let the combination cool in the fridge for at least 2 to 12 hours.

Pull out the ice cream combination from the fridge and stir a few times.

Mount the frozen ice cream maker bowl and pour the mixture into it.

Connect the machine, then press ice cream and the start button.

When the cycle is over, transfer the ice cream to an airtight freezer-safe container or serve right away. If you like a harder consistency, allow the ice cream to freeze for 2 hours or more before serving.

Nutrition:

- Calories: 435
- Fat: 18g
- Carbs: 69g
- Sugar: 68g
- Protein: 3g
- Sodium: 356mg

48. Strawberry and Coconut Ice Cream

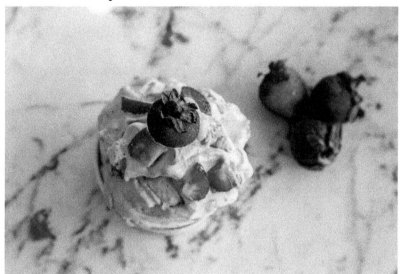

Preparation Time: 25 Minutes

Cooking Time: 0 Minutes

Servings: 8

Ingredients:

- 1 Cup whole milk
- 3 Cups strawberries, cut in halves
- ¾ Cup powdered sugar
- 1 ½ Cups heavy cream
- ½ Cup coconut milk
- 1 Teaspoon vanilla extract

Directions:

Freeze the ice cream maker bowl rendering to manufacturer instructions, frequently 12 to 24 hours.

In the machine, add the strawberries, milk, and powdered sugar.

Blitz until you get a smooth and creamy mixture. Blend for about 3 minutes.

Pour the mixture into a bowl and stir in the vanilla extract, coconut milk, and heavy cream. Mix until combined.

Cover the mixture with plastic wrap and let the mixture cool in the refrigerator for at least 2 to 12 hours.

Pull out the ice cream mixture from the refrigerator and stir a few times.

Install the frozen ice cream maker bowl and pour the mixture into the ice cream maker.

Connect the machine and press ice cream and the start button.

When the cycle is finished, transfer the ice cream to an airtight freezer-safe container or serve right away. The ice cream will be soft and creamy. If you like a harder texture, allow the ice cream to freeze for 2 hours or more before serving.

Nutrition:

- Calories: 386
- Fat: 26g
- Carbs: 37g
- Sugar: 32g
- Protein: 4g
- Sodium: 47mg

49. Almond Coconut Ice Cream

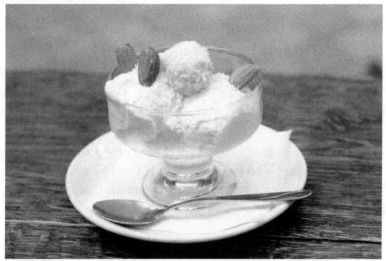

Preparation Time: 25 Minutes

Cooking Time: 0 Minutes

Servings: 8

Ingredients:

- 1 Cup whole milk
- ¾ Cup powdered sugar
- 2 Teaspoons vanilla extract
- ¼ Cup crushed almonds
- ½ Cup coconut flakes
- 2 Cups heavy cream

Directions:

Freeze the ice cream maker bowl rendering to manufacturer directions, usually 12 to 24 hours.

Meanwhile, in a large mixing bowl, add the milk, heavy cream, and powdered sugar.

Add the vanilla extract and mix until everything is combined.

Cover the combination with plastic wrap and let the combination cool in the fridge for at least 2 to 12 hours.

Pull out the ice cream combination from the fridge and stir a few times.

Install the frozen ice cream maker container, then pour the combination into it.

Connect the machine, then press ice cream and the start button.

Around 5 minutes before the end of the churning process, add the crushed almonds and coconut little by little into the ice cream and let it mix in.

When the cycle is over, transfer the ice cream to an airtight freezer-safe container or serve right away. If you like a harder consistency, allow the ice cream to freeze for 2 hours or more before serving.

Nutrition:

- Calories: 612
- Fat: 48g
- Carbs: 37g
- Sugar: 28g
- Protein: 13g
- Sodium: 48mg

50. Easy Vanilla Ice Cream

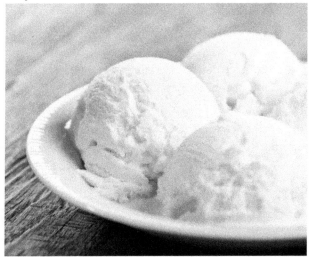

Preparation Time: 25 Minutes

Cooking Time: 0 Minutes

Servings: 8

Ingredients:

- ¾ Cup granulated sugar
- 2 Cup heavy whipping cream
- 1 Cup milk
- 2 Teaspoons vanilla extract

Directions:

Freeze the ice cream maker bowl rendering to manufacturer instructions, usually 12 to 24 hours.

Meanwhile, in a large saucepan, add the whole milk, heavy cream, and sugar. Stir to combine.

Over medium-low heat, bring the combination to a soft simmering and constantly whisk until the sugar is completely dissolved, about 10-12 minutes.

Pour the mixture into a clean bowl, preferably with a spout. Stir in the vanilla extract and let cool to room temperature.

Cover thru plastic wrap and place in the fridge for at least 2 to 12 hours.

Pull out the ice cream combination from the fridge and stir a few times.

Install the frozen ice cream maker bowl, then pour the combination into the ice cream maker. Attach the machine and press ice cream and the start button.

When the cycle is over, transfer the ice cream to an airtight freezer-safe container or serve right away. If you like a harder texture, let the ice cream freeze for 2 hours or more before serving.

Nutrition:

- Calories: 311 Fat: 14g
- Carbs: 45g
- Sugar: 43g
- Protein: 5g
- Sodium: 69mg

Conclusion

Thank you for reaching the end of this book. I hope that by now, you exactly must know how to use your Yonanas Frozen Treat Maker and had tried several recipes already.

Pro tips to make perfect soft-serve dessert

Here are some pro tips to make a perfect soft-serve dessert:

1. Freeze a tub of coconut milk overnight, and then scoop out the solid part into your Yonanas machine.
2. Try using different frozen fruits, like mangoes or pears.
3. Add in banana to sweeten your soft-serve dessert if you want.
4. If your fruit puree is too thick, add in honey or agave nectar and some water to thin it up.
5. Add in some instant-dissolving
6. Stevia-based sugar to increase sweetness.
7. Add some finely chopped nuts to your soft-serve dessert if you want a nutty flavor to it.
8. Use coconut vanilla extract as flavoring instead of vanilla extract, and mix it with equal parts water and sugar for the perfect consistency of your soft-serve dessert.
9. There is no need to cool your Yonanas machine before making your dessert since it uses the tub of coconut milk you chilled and took out earlier.

When you're making different kinds of soft-serve desserts, here are some additional tips:

1. Freeze a tub of coconut milk overnight, and then scoop out the solid part into your Yonanas machine.
2. Add in yogurt if you want to flavor it with a cheese flavor. You can also use Greek yogurt or kefir instead if that's what you're more familiar with.

3. You can add sugar, honey, agave nectar, or any sweeteners you like into your soft-serve dessert.

4. Add any instant-dissolving stevia-based sugar to increase sweetness. However, don't use too much of it since it is calorie-free. It is also better to gradually increase the sweetness level than to dump a lot of sweeteners at once. The reason for this is because the more sweetener you add to the mixture, the waterier your soft-serve dessert will become. You might eventually lose the creamy texture.

5. If you want to add flavor to your soft-serve dessert, there are several ways you can do it. You can experiment with adding vanilla extract, cinnamon powder, or any other flavors you like. You can also use coconut vanilla extract since Vanilla and coconut seem to go well together.

6. If the consistency of your soft-serve dessert is too thick for your liking, add in some water or milk (regular milk works best). Remember that too much liquid will thin down your soft-serve dessert too much and will eventually lose that creamy texture it has to begin with.

Yonanas Frozen Treat Maker is a great investment if you are a fan of homemade soft-serve desserts. And one of the reasons I like this product so much is that it's just so easy to use. You just open up the frozen tub of coconut milk, scoop out any solid part, add in ice and the ingredients (if any) in your Yonanas machine, and then press the Start timer button to get your frozen dessert. If needed, you may also add in extra water or ice to get your desired consistency.

If you are the type of person that enjoys eating fruit for dessert, then this product is definitely for you. It is easy to use, and the frozen soft-serve dessert it makes tastes very good. If you're on a diet, then this is definitely an excellent treat to help quench your sweet tooth instead of having a full-sized dessert.

Another thing I like about this machine is that it has a smooth soft-serve texture compared to other homemade frozen desserts like sorbets and ice cream, which tend to be icy and grainy. Remember these reasons to inspire you.

Again, thank you and enjoy your frozen treats.

CPSIA information can be obtained
at www.ICGtesting.com
Printed in the USA
BVHW012329150321
602550BV00005B/601

9 781802 161434